OUTBREAK!

TYPHOID
EPIDEMIC

KENNY ABDO

Fly!
An Imprint of Abdo Zoom
abdobooks.com

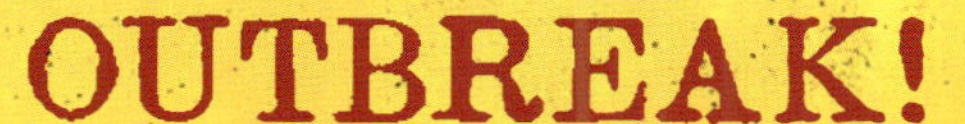

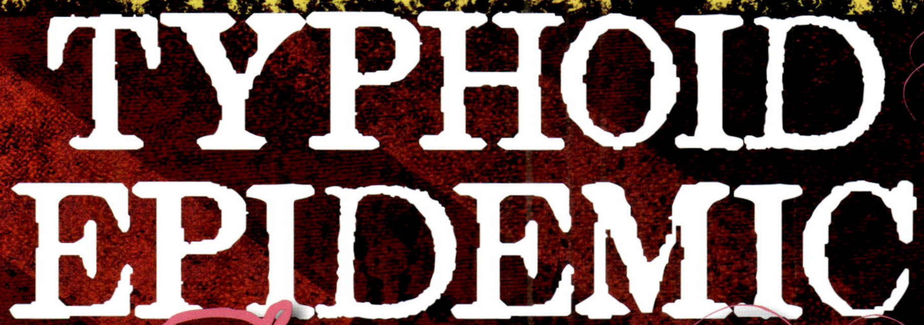

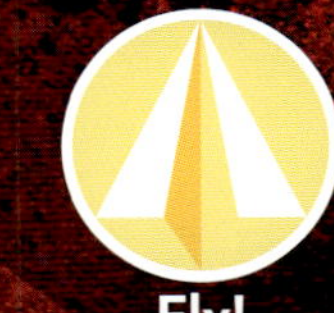

abdobooks.com

Published by Abdo Zoom, a division of ABDO, P.O. Box 398166, Minneapolis, Minnesota 55439. Copyright © 2021 by Abdo Consulting Group, Inc. International copyrights reserved in all countries. No part of this book may be reproduced in any form without written permission from the publisher. Fly!™ is a trademark and logo of Abdo Zoom.

Printed in the United States of America, North Mankato, Minnesota.
102020
012021

Photo Credits: Alamy, AP Images, Everett Collection, Library of Congress, Science Source, Shutterstock, ©National Museum of Health and Medicine p16 / CC BY 2.0
Production Contributors: Kenny Abdo, Jennie Forsberg, Grace Hansen
Design Contributors: Dorothy Toth, Neil Klinepier, Laura Graphenteen

Library of Congress Control Number: 2020910909

Publisher's Cataloging-in-Publication Data

Names: Abdo, Kenny, author.
Title: Typhoid epidemic / by Kenny Abdo
Description: Minneapolis, Minnesota : Abdo Zoom, 2021 | Series: Outbreak! | Includes online resources and index.
Identifiers: ISBN 9781098223304 (lib. bdg.) | ISBN 9781098224004 (ebook) | ISBN 9781098224356 (Read-to-Me ebook)
Subjects: LCSH: Typhoid fever--Juvenile literature. | Enteric fever--Juvenile literature. | Epidemics--Juvenile literature. | Epidemics--History--Juvenile literature. | Plague--History--Juvenile literature.
Classification: DDC 614.49--dc23

TABLE OF CONTENTS

Typhoid Epidemic 4

Symptoms...................... 8

Source 10

Outbreak! 14

Glossary 22

Online Resources 23

Index 24

TYPHOID EPIDEMIC

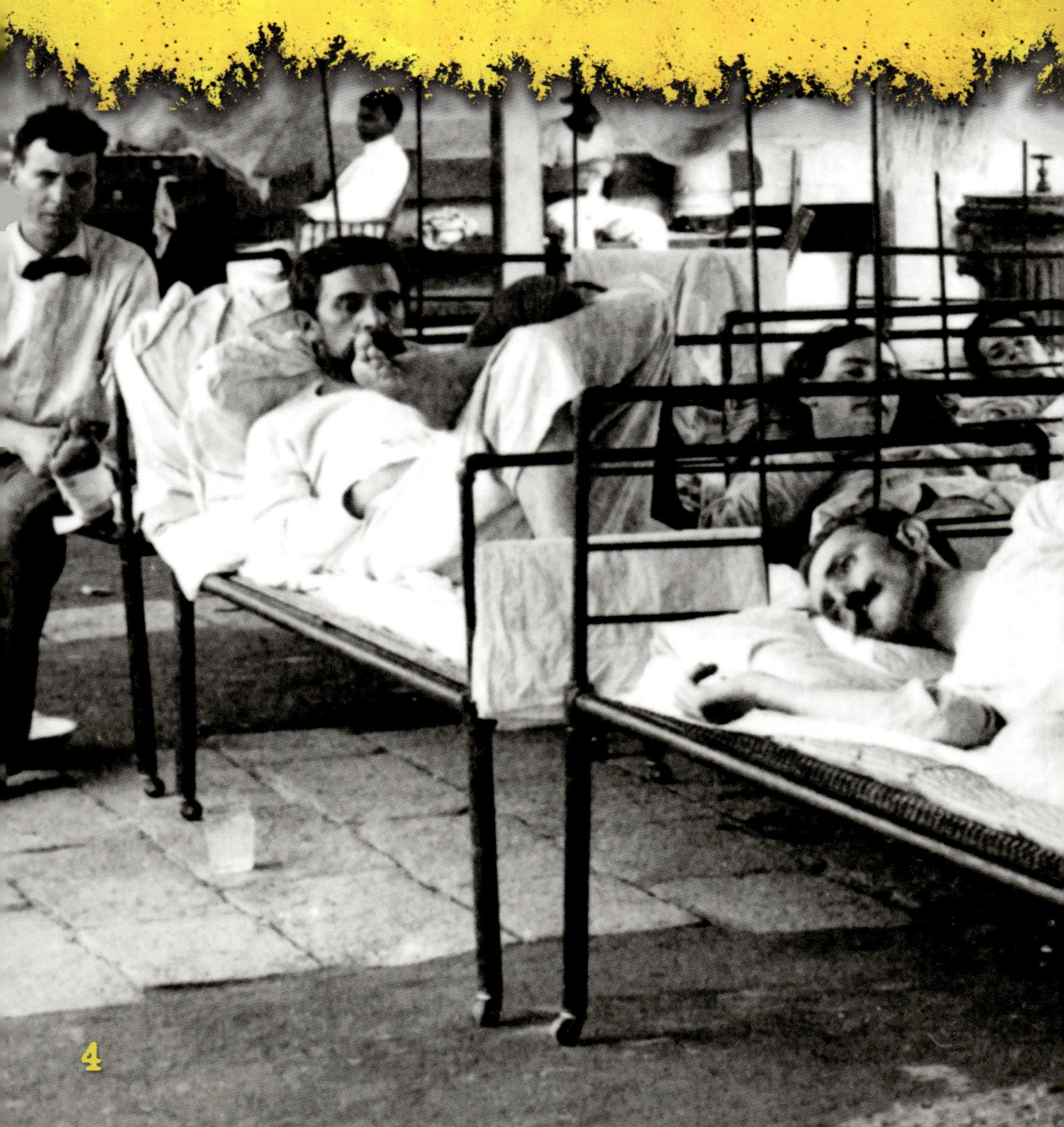

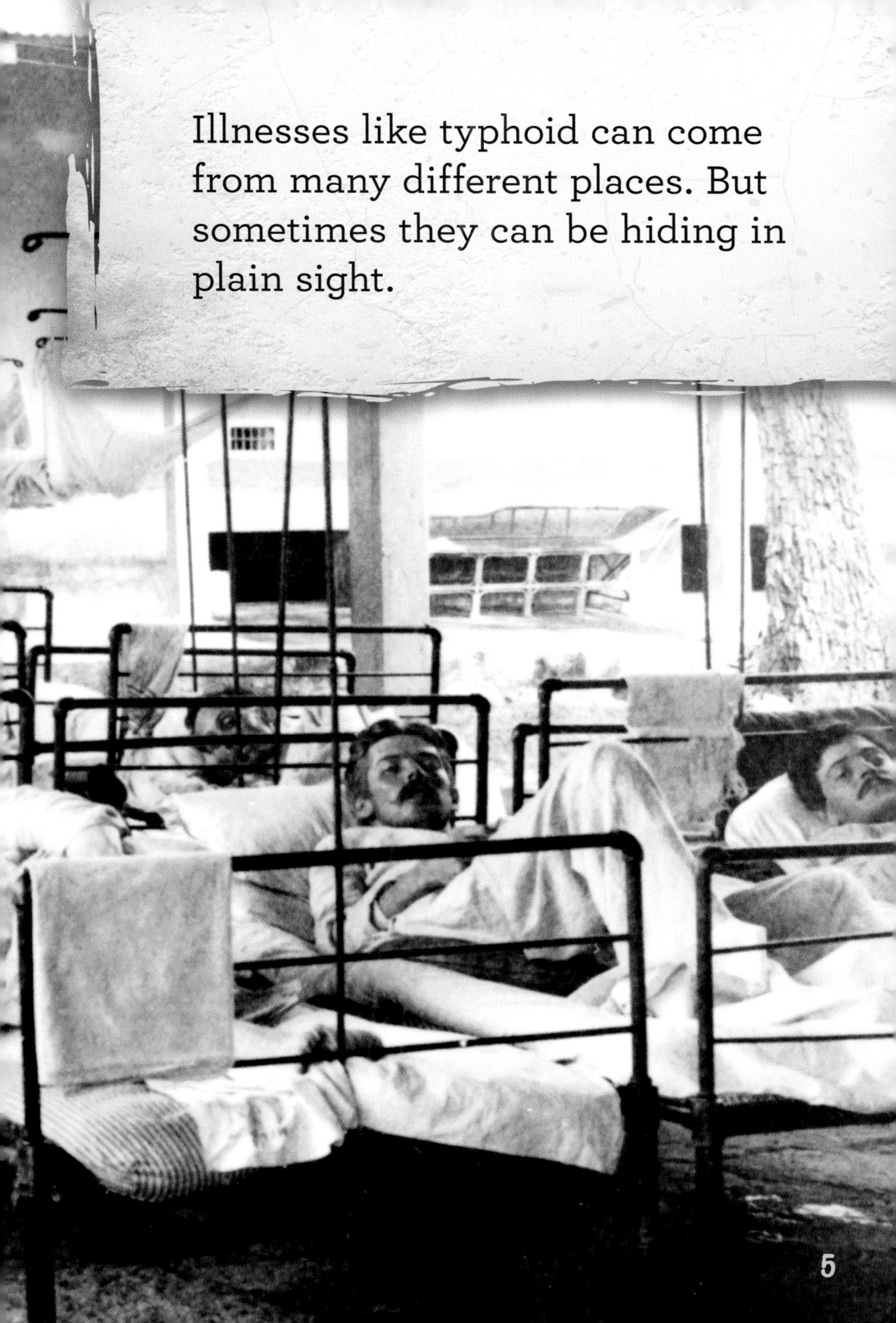

Illnesses like typhoid can come from many different places. But sometimes they can be hiding in plain sight.

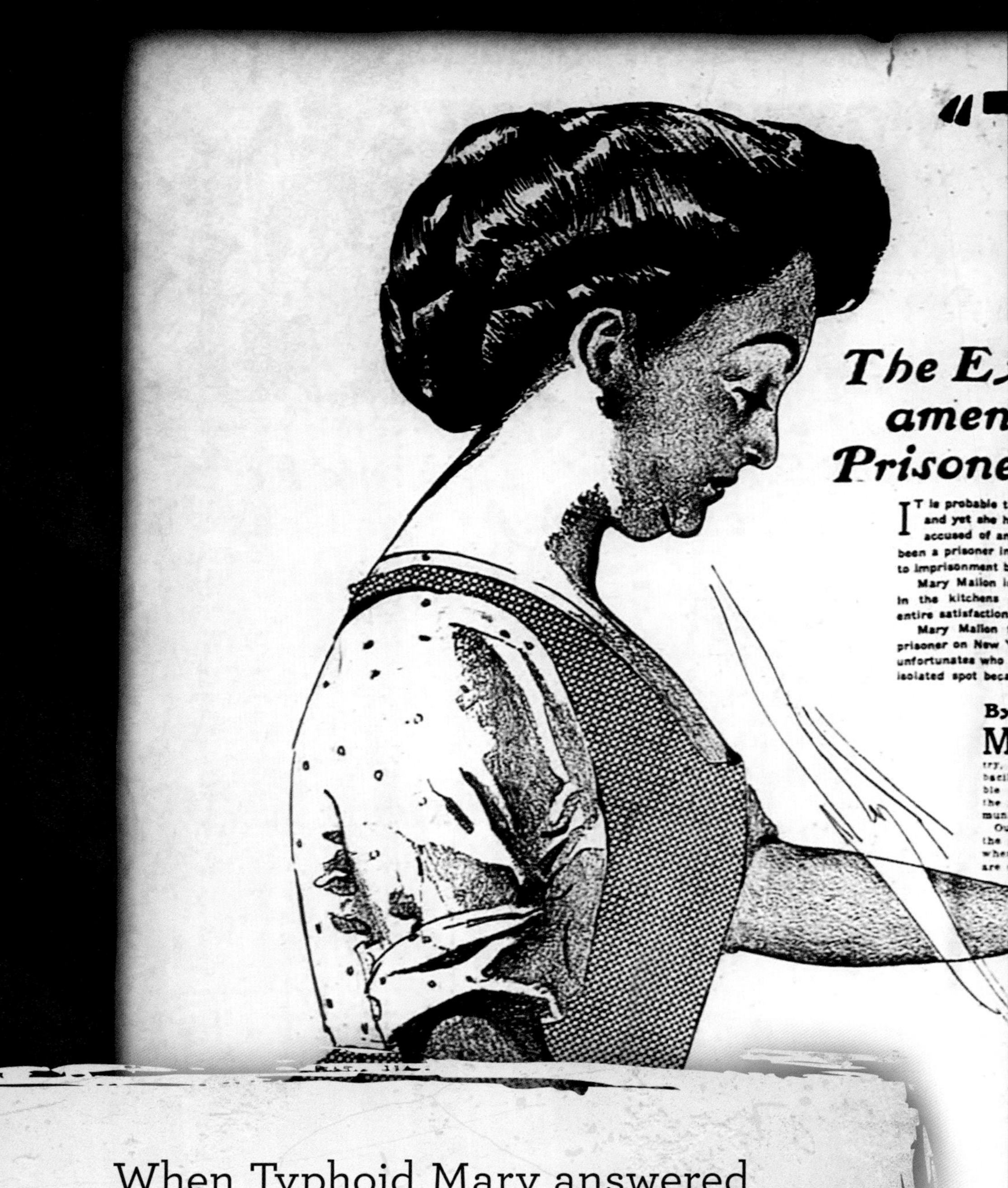

When Typhoid Mary answered
a help wanted ad, she had no
idea she was a carrier of one of
history's most infectious diseases.

TYPHOID MARY"

...raordinary Predic-
...f Mary Mallon, a
...on New York's Quarantine Hospita...

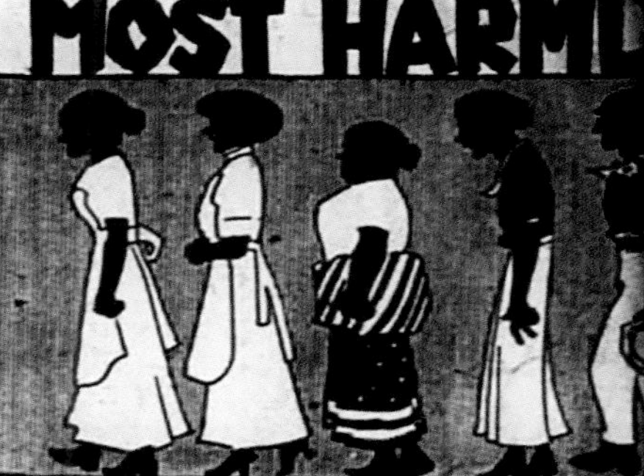

4 Laundresses.

Mallon is a prisoner for life—
...itted no crime, has never been
...or wicked act, and has never
...t, nor has she been sentenced
...ge.
...by profession. She has served
...New York millionaires with
... years.
...than two years has been a
...arantine island, along with the
...time to time removed to this
...are suffering from smallpox.

scarlet fever or other contagious diseases.

But while Mary sees these unfortunate victims of various diseases come on the hospital boat and, in due time, return to their homes and friends—Mary stays on forever.

There is probably in the whole wide world no prisoner that can furnish a parallel to the extreme misfortune which has brought Mary Mallon to North Brother Island. Through no fault of hers, Mary Mallon is a living, walking incubator of typhoid fever germs. Every day for two years the officials of the New York Board of Health have examined Mary, and they have been discouraged to find a bountiful supply of new typhoid fever bacilli freshly

made each twenty-four hours by Mary...
Mary Mallon, in the five years befor...
authorities got their hands on her, wa...
of twenty-six cases of typhoid fever...
others. So far as is known, the woma...
had the disease, and is not now sick w...
But somewhere in her anatomy, perha...
of the gall duct, there is a never faili...
typhoid fever germs. To the positi...
Board of Health Mary has been gene...
typhoid bacilli for seven years. This...
they are able to trace her history...

Wm. H. Parks, New York Board of Health.

...ALLON is the chief of fifty persons,
... of whom have been discovered
... the past two years, in this coun-
...know in medical science as typhus
.... Her case is the most remarka-
...ch we are acquainted, because of
...f persons to whom she has com-
... disease.
...f the case leads us to believe that
...erms lodge in the gall bladder,
...ive indefinitely. From there they
...rough the body by the bile.

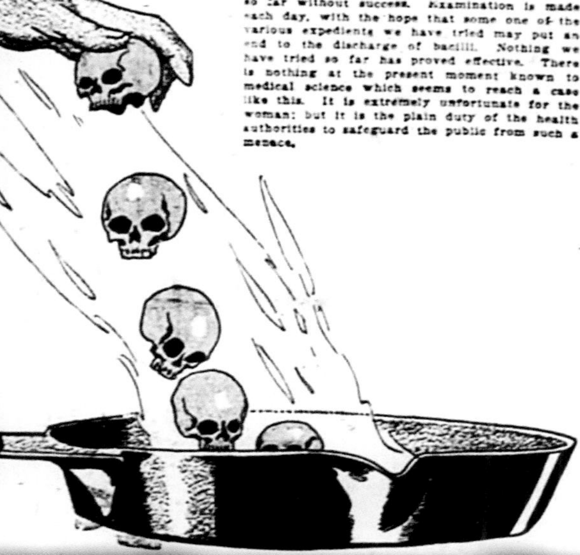

She is confined on North Brother Island, where she has been a prisoner for two years, and where, of course, she will remain indefinitely. She is a large, healthy looking woman, a typical cook, and there is nothing in her outward appearance to indicate that she is other than normal. She is, of course, segregated with the typhoid patients. When we consider that she has been spreading the contagion for many years, it is clear that she will be a prisoner on North Brother Island for a long time, perhaps for life; certainly until we are convinced that the typhus germs and typhus tendencies have been eliminated from her body.

Every effort has been made by the health authorities to cure the unfortunate woman, but so far without success. Examination is made each day, with the hope that some one of the various expedients we have tried may put an end to the discharge of bacilli. Nothing we have tried so far has proved effective. There is nothing at the present moment known to medical science which seems to reach a case like this. It is extremely unfortunate for the woman; but it is the plain duty of the health authorities to safeguard the public from such a menace.

The Extraordi...
and Dis...

The Official ...

IN the Winter of 1906 I was called on to investigate a household epidemic of typhoid fever which had broken out in the latter part of August at Oyster Bay, N. Y. The epidemic had been studied carefully immediately after it took place, but its cause had not been ascertained with as much certainty as seemed desirable to the owner of the property.

The essential facts concerning the investigation follow:

At Oyster Bay, in the Summer of 1906, six persons in a household of eleven were attacked with typhoid fever. The house was large, surrounded with ample grounds, in a desirable part of the village, and had been rented for the Summer by a New York banker.

The first person was taken sick on August 27 and the last on September 3. The diagnosis of typhoid was positive. Two of the patients were sent to the Nassau Hospital at Mineola. The others were attended by capable physicians at Oyster Bay. None of the subsequent cases apparently resulted from the first, although the interval from the first to the last might permit of this assumption. But whether the disease was transmitted from one person to another after the first case occurred was not a matter of great consequence. The most important question was how the first case occurred.

Germ Source a Mystery.

Typhoid fever is an unusual disease in Oyster Bay, according to the three physicians who share the medical practise there. At the time of the outbreak no other case was known. None followed.

The milk supply of this house was the same as used by most of the other persons in the village, all of whom remained well. The cream also was from a source which supplied several other families in the vicinity.

To the first investigators it seemed that the water must have been contaminated. They were

SYMPTOMS

Typhoid, or typhoid fever, starts with a high fever. People will feel weak and have stomach pains and headaches. A rash of red spots can also develop.

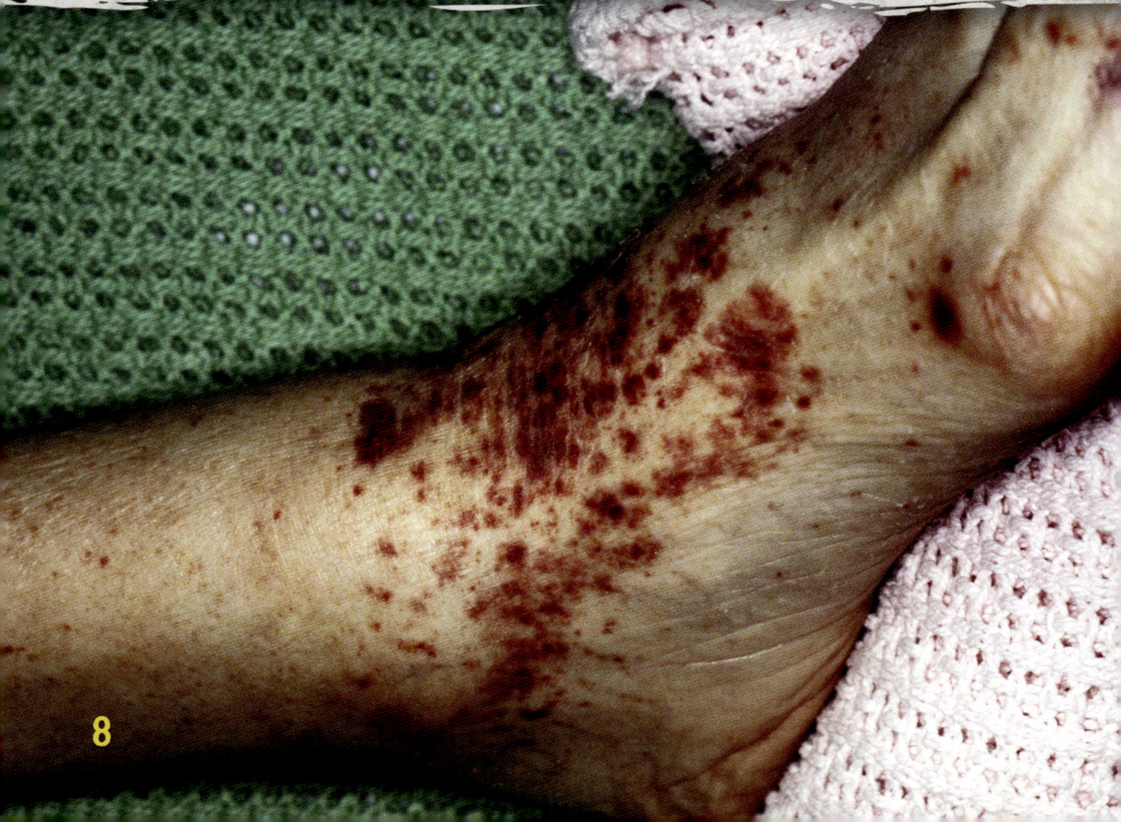

Without treatment, victims become **delirious**. They also lie motionless from exhaustion. This is known as the typhoid state.

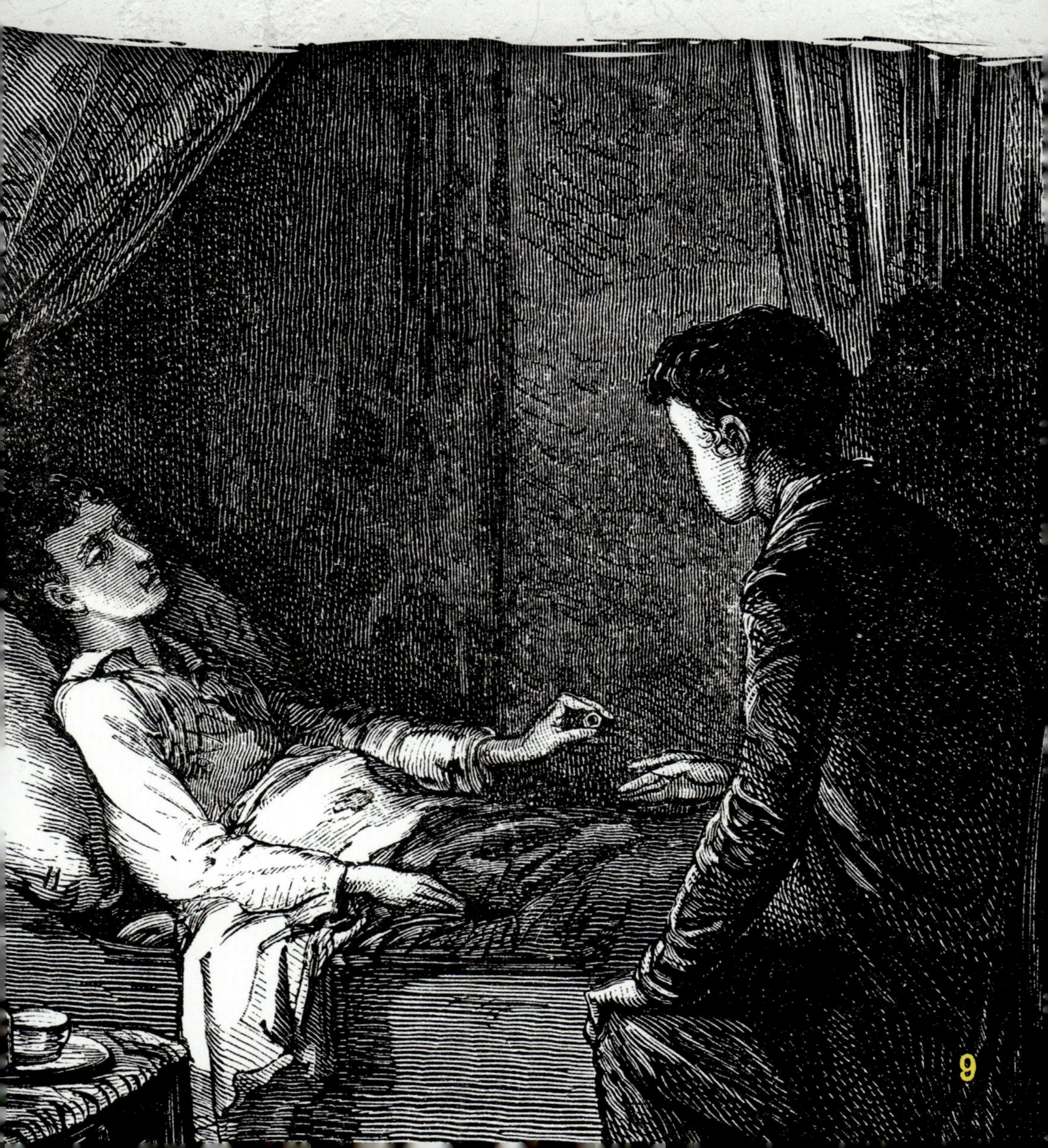

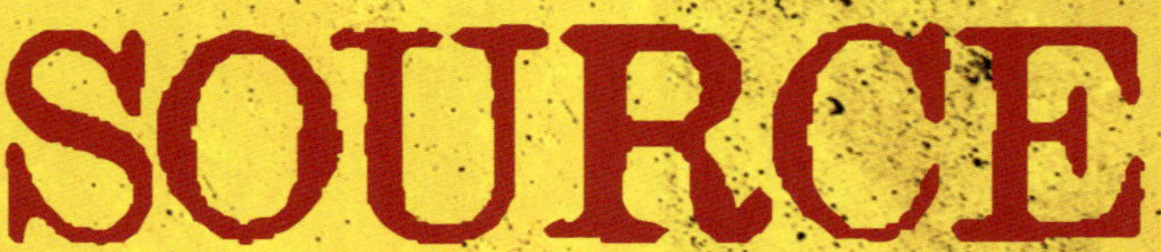

Typhoid fever is caused by *Salmonella* typhi bacteria. *Salmonella* comes from the intestines of animals. It is a serious health threat, especially to children.

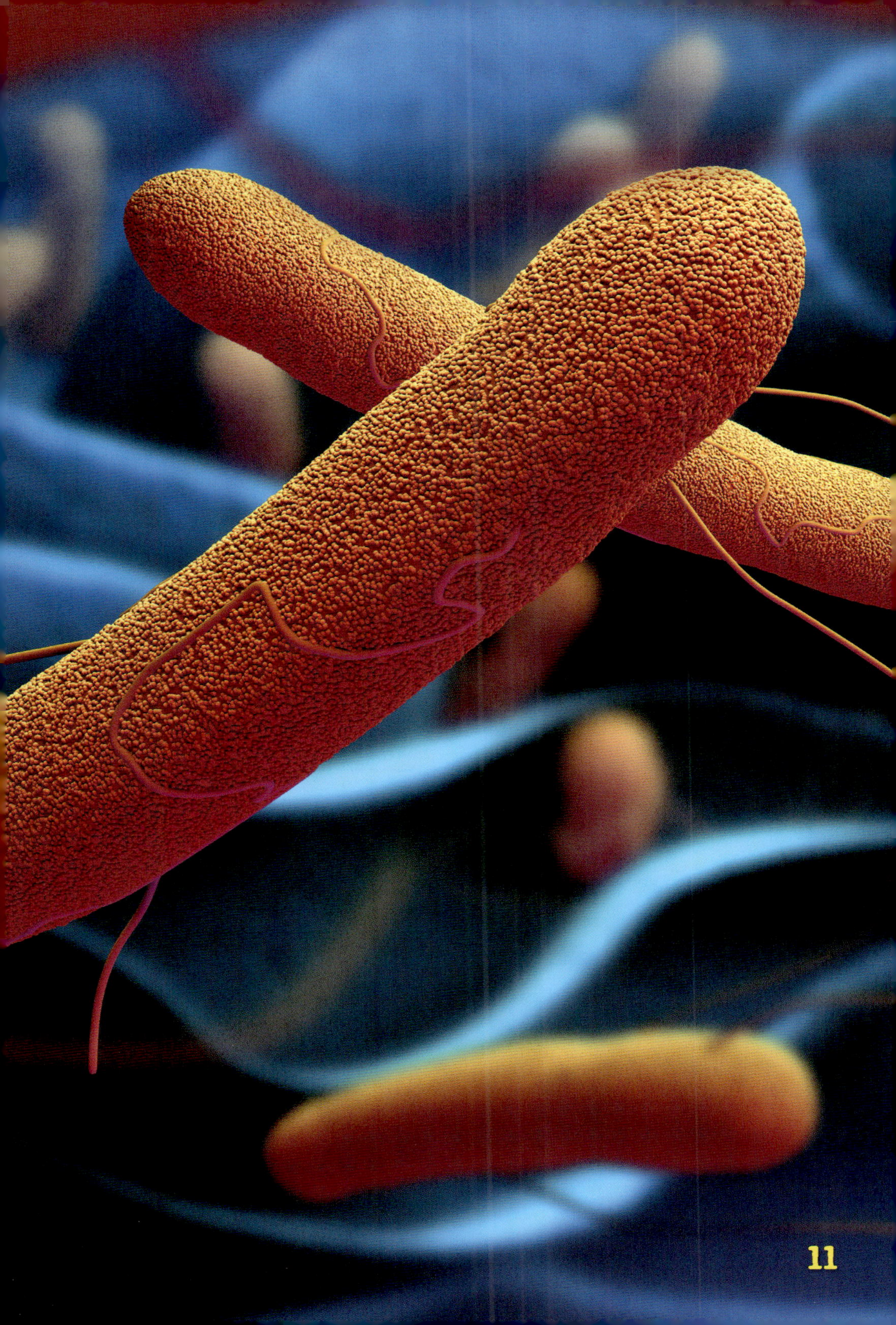

New-York Tribune.

ILLUSTRATED SUPPLEMENT.

SUNDAY, MARCH 8, 1903.

THE TYPHOID GERM HUNTERS ARE AFTER THE MEN WHO CUT ICE FROM POLLUTED WATERS TO SELL IN NEW-YORK

(Photograph by O'Neil & Langley.)

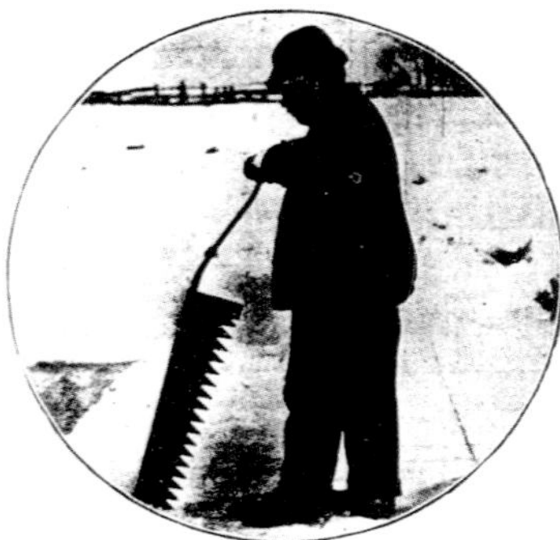

SAWING THE BLOCKS.

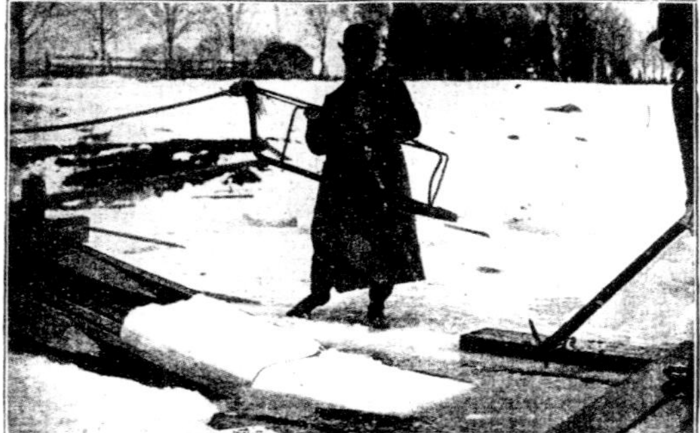

READY TO THROW THE CRADLE ON THE ICE BLOCKS.

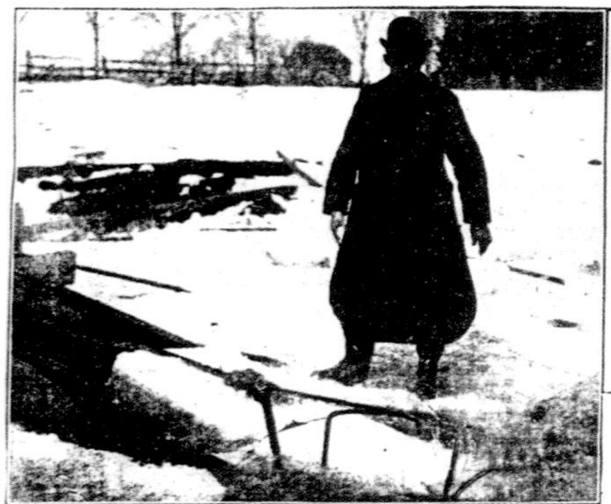

THE CRADLE GRIPS THE CAKES AND HOISTING BEGINS.

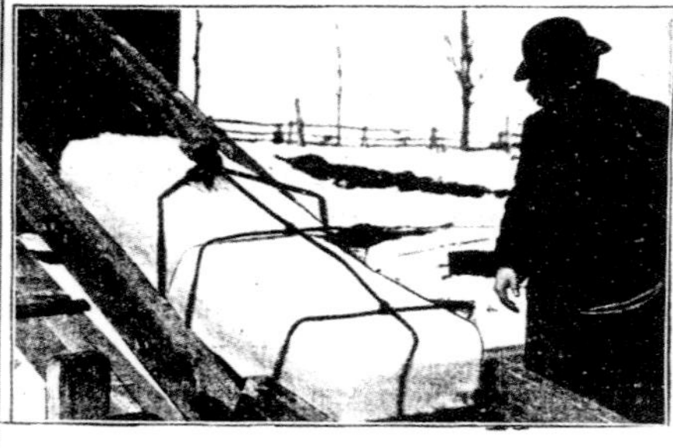

ICE BLOCKS GOING UP THE SLIDE.

ICE BLOCK JUST READY TO FALL INTO ICEHOUSE.

HOW THE CAKES ARE PACKED IN THE ICEHOUSE.

Typhoid fever spreads through **contaminated** food and water. Close contact with someone who is **infected** also **transmits** it.

TYPHOID FEVER

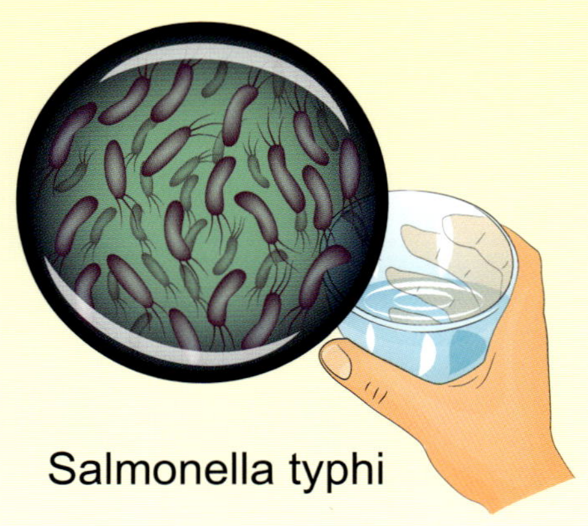

Salmonella typhi

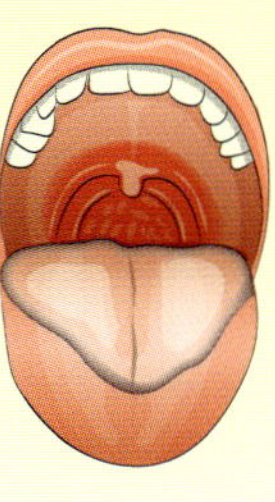

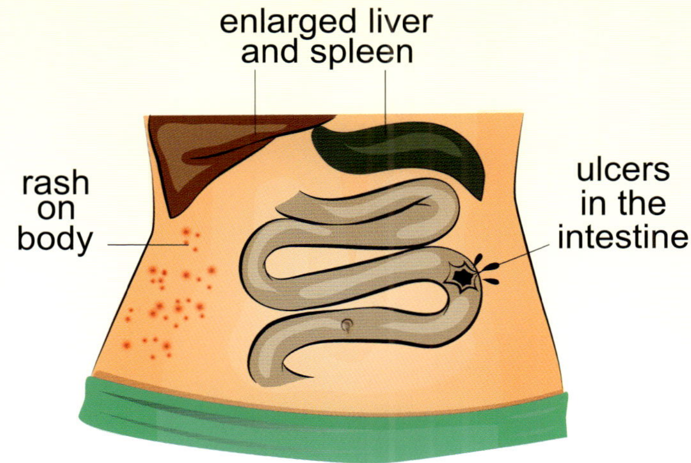

OUTBREAK!

Born in 1869 Northern Ireland, Mary Mallon immigrated to New York in 1883. Wanting to start a new life, she found work as an inhouse servant for wealthy families.

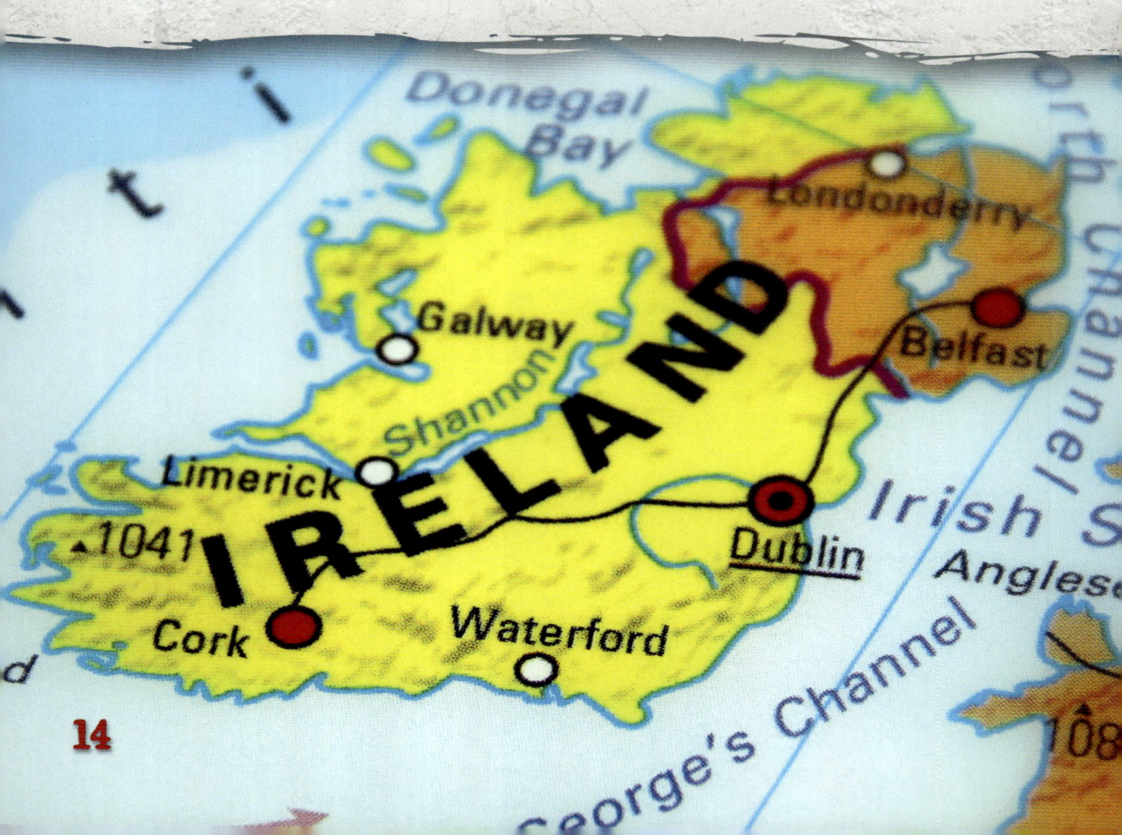

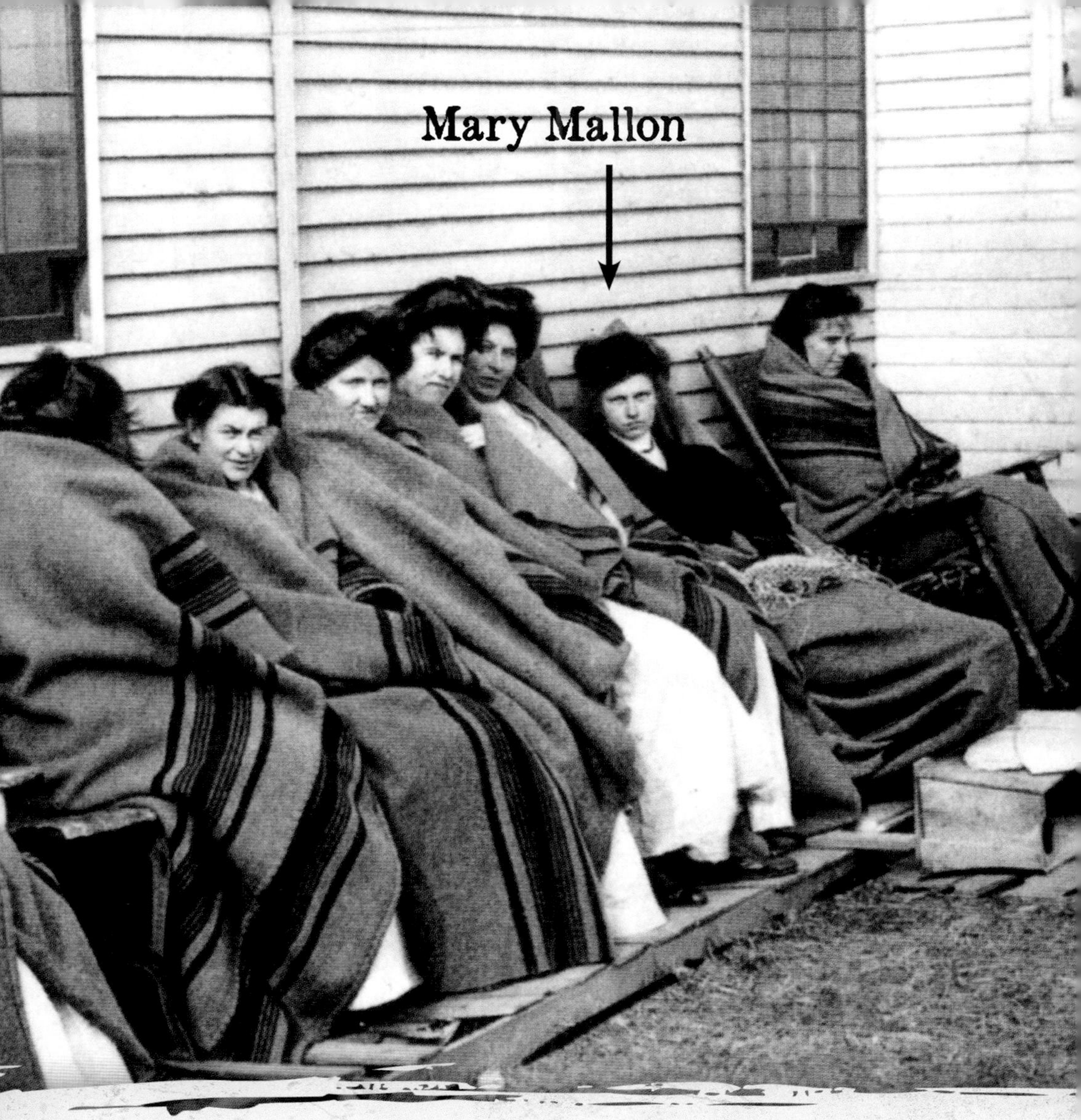

In 1906, six people staying with banker Charles Warren contracted typhoid. Sanitary engineer George Soper investigated, revealing the source. It was Mallon, Warren's cook.

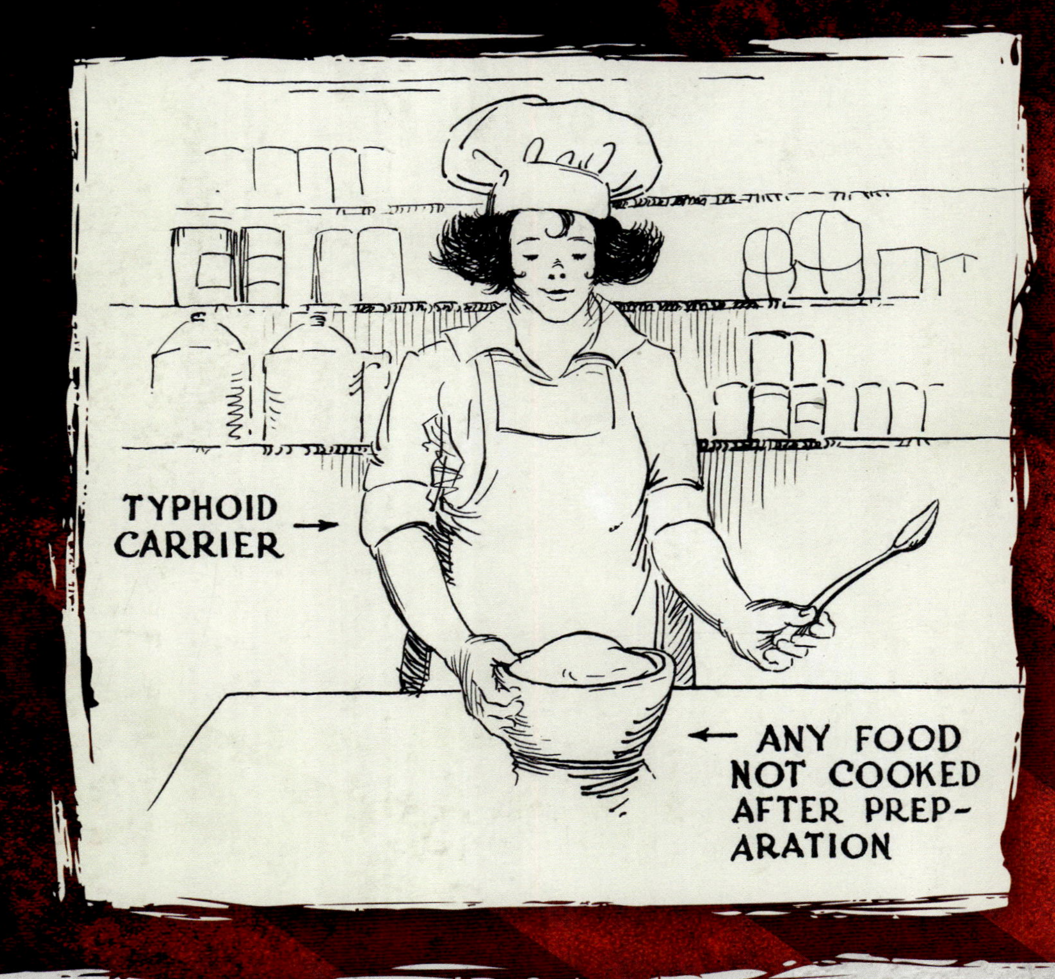

There were no regular **sanitation** practices at that time, so the illness was common. There were multiple outbreaks in New York. Mallon was **asymptomatic**. Soper found that seven families she had worked for also reported cases of typhoid.

Mallon was believed to have **infected** 51 people. Three of the infected died. She was taken into custody in 1907 for three years.

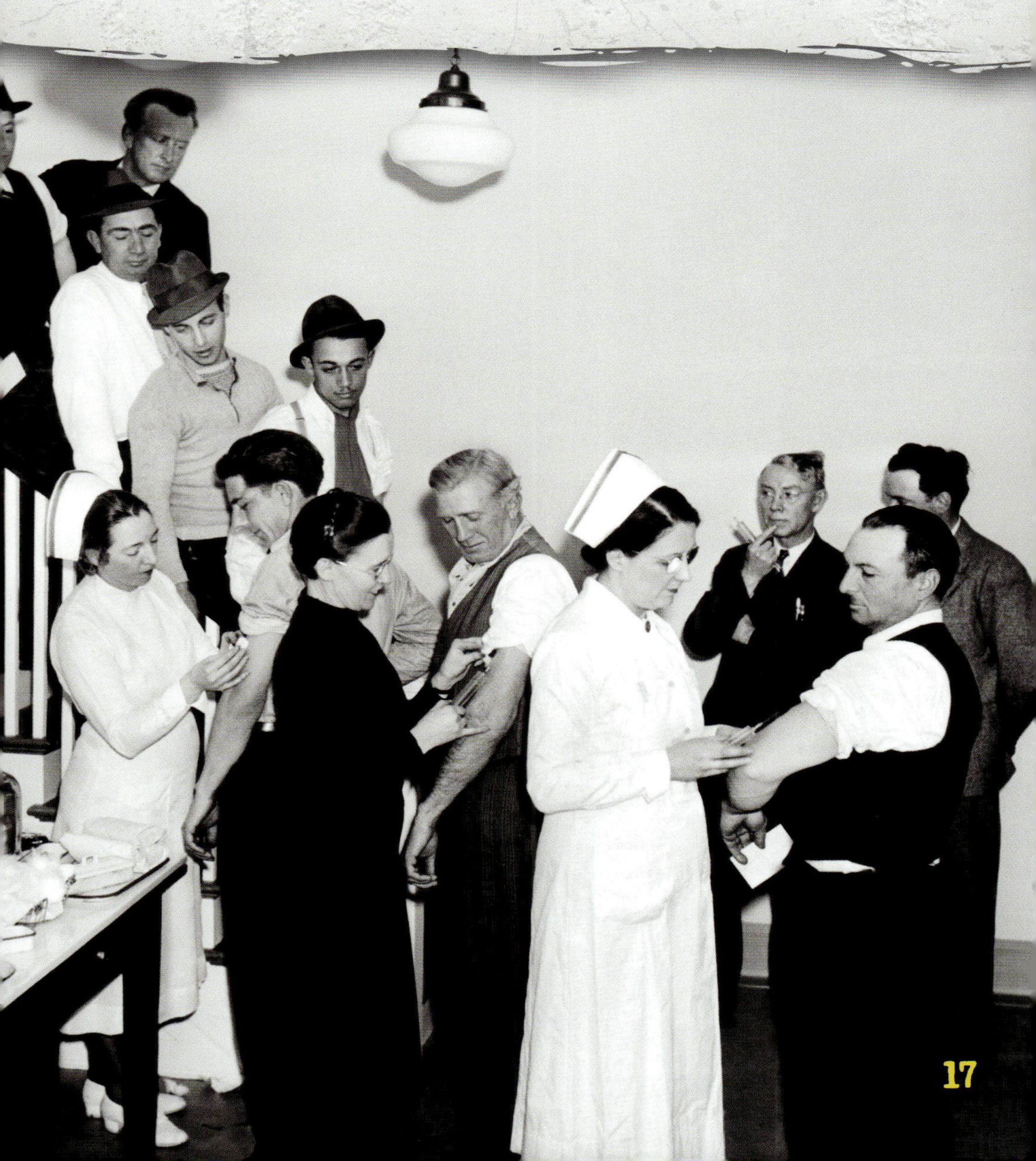

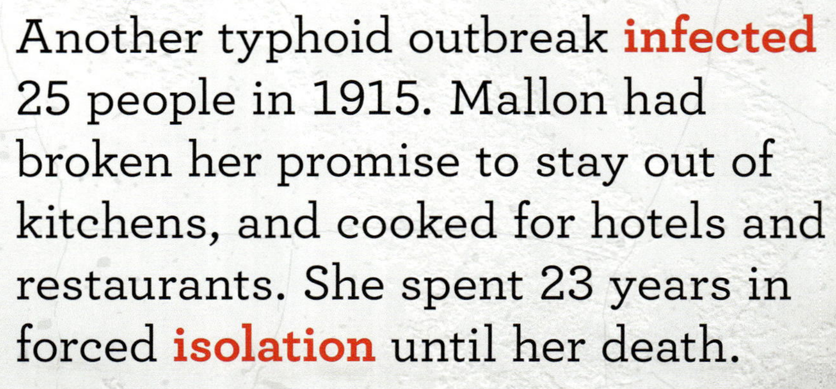

Another typhoid outbreak **infected** 25 people in 1915. Mallon had broken her promise to stay out of kitchens, and cooked for hotels and restaurants. She spent 23 years in forced **isolation** until her death.

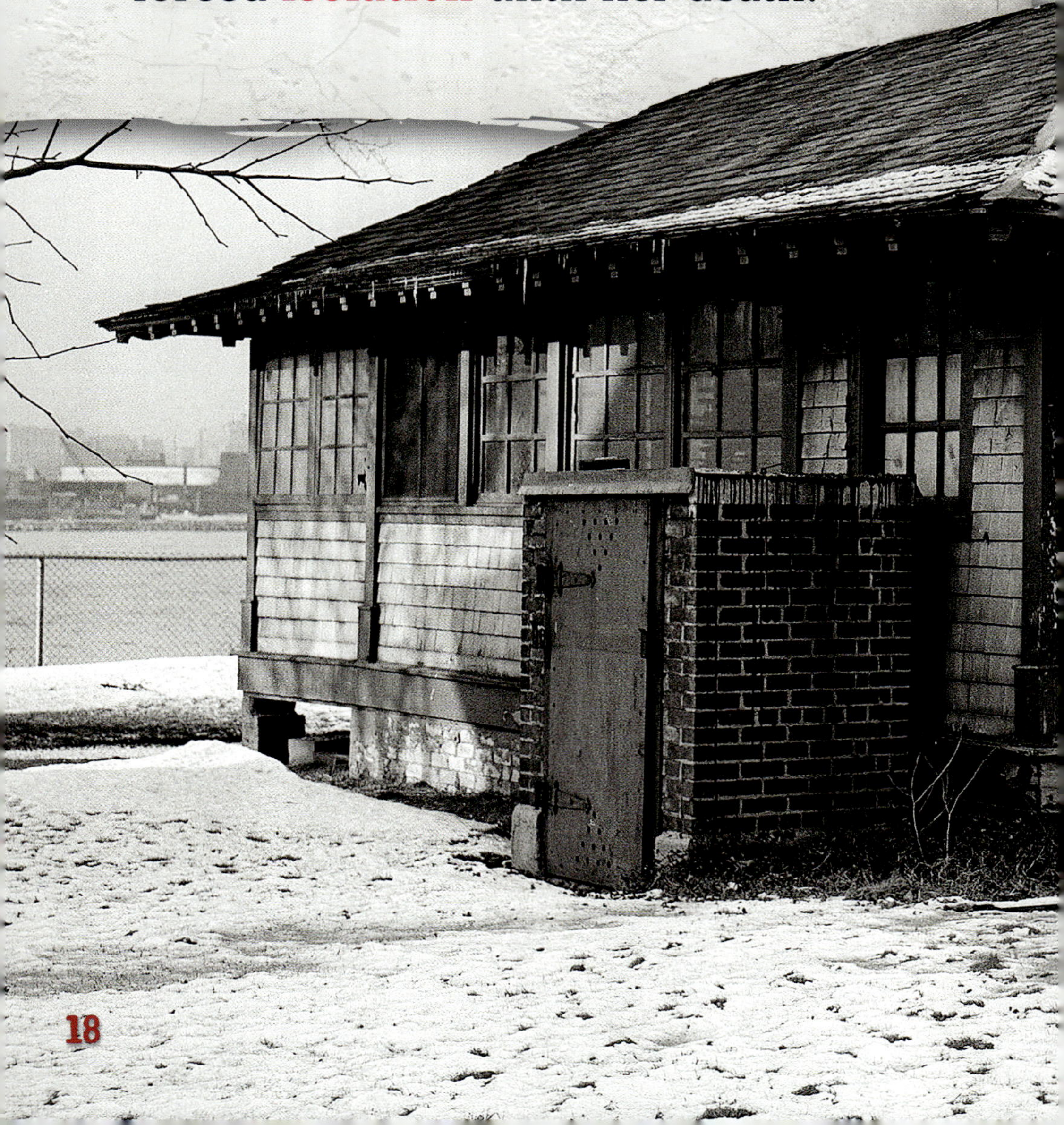

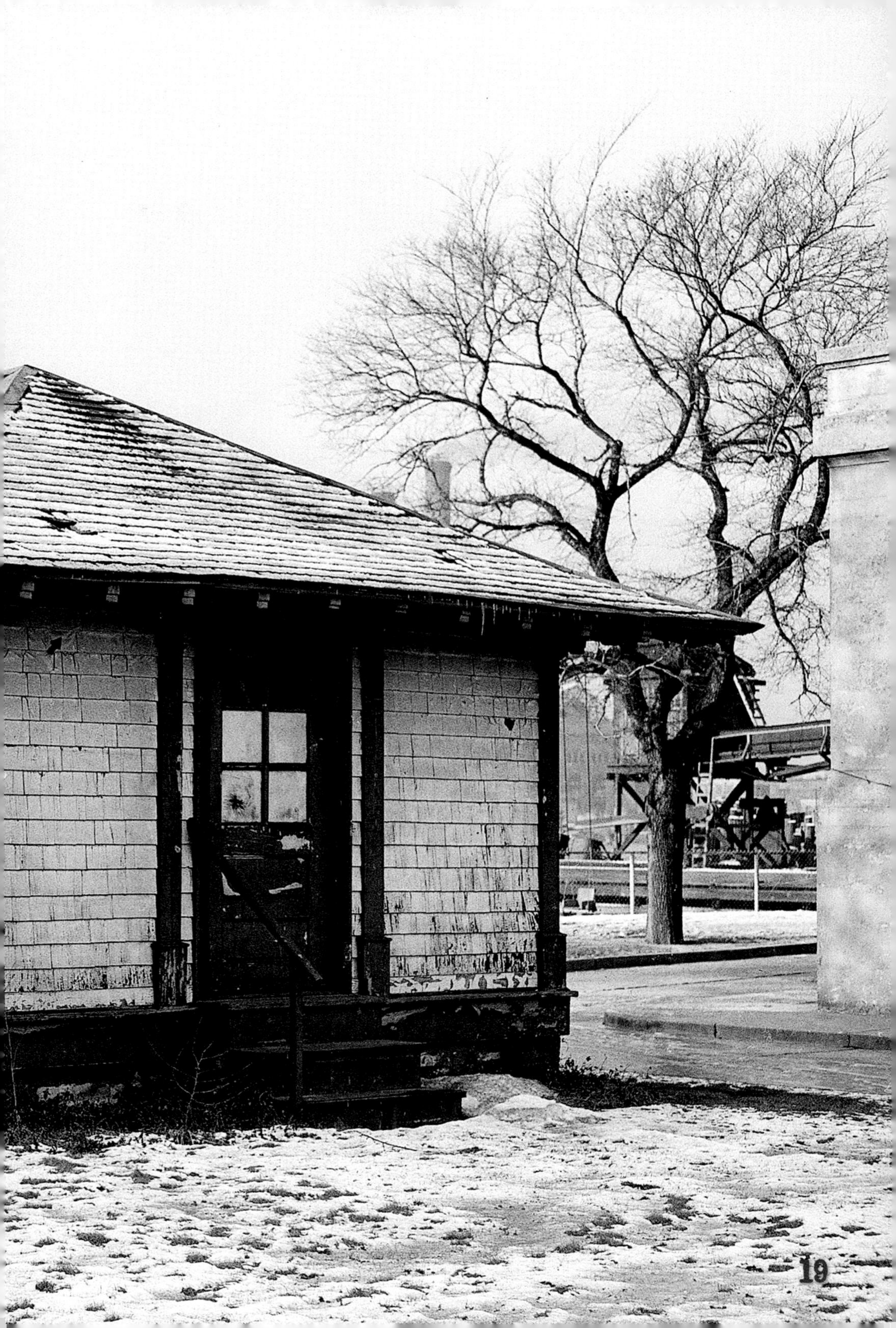

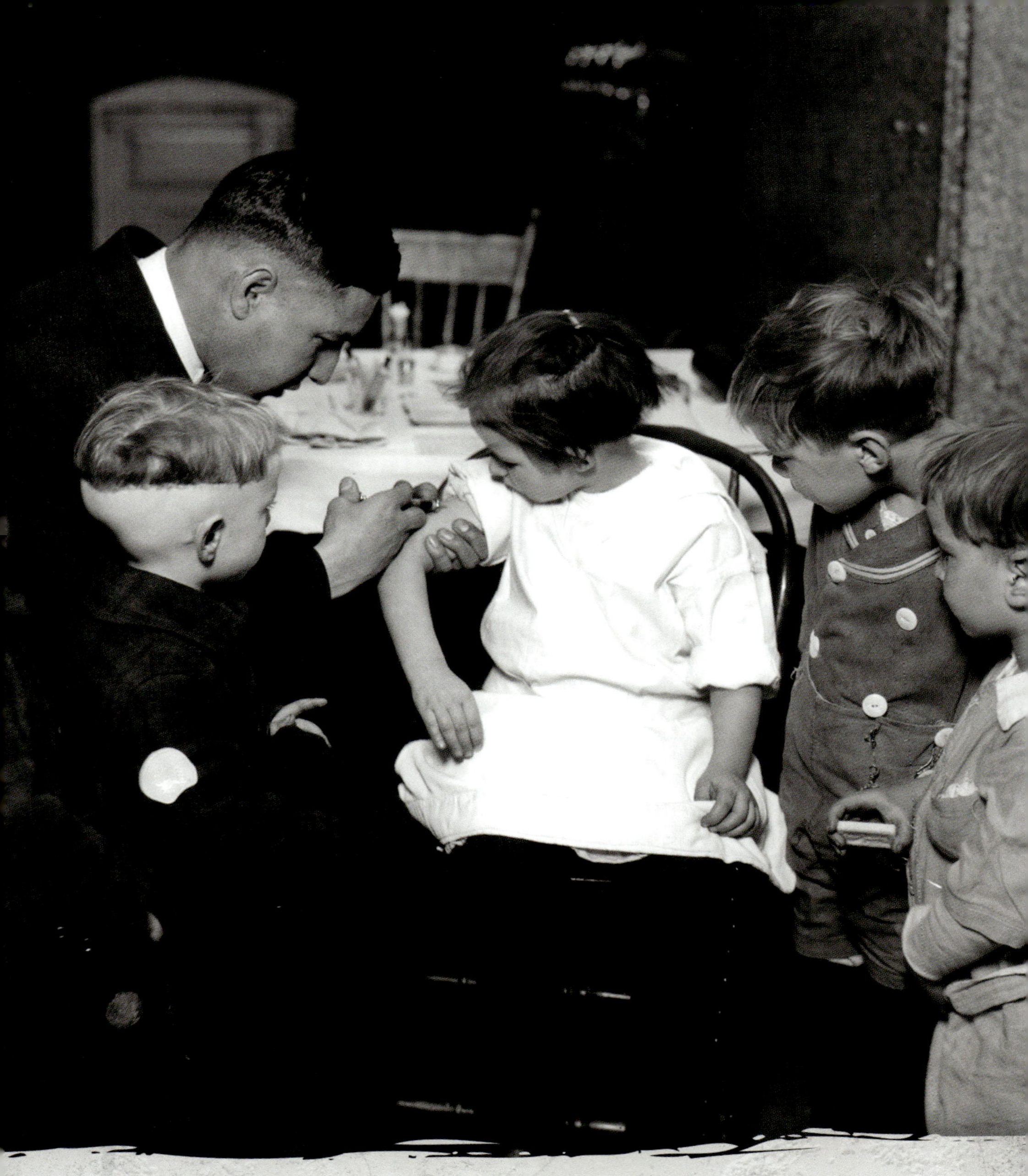

A **vaccine** for typhoid was developed in 1896. It was made available to the public in 1914.

Today typhoid still rages on. Up to 20 million people get sick from typhoid each year. So, it is best to wash hands often, eat properly cooked food, and make sure drinking water is clean.

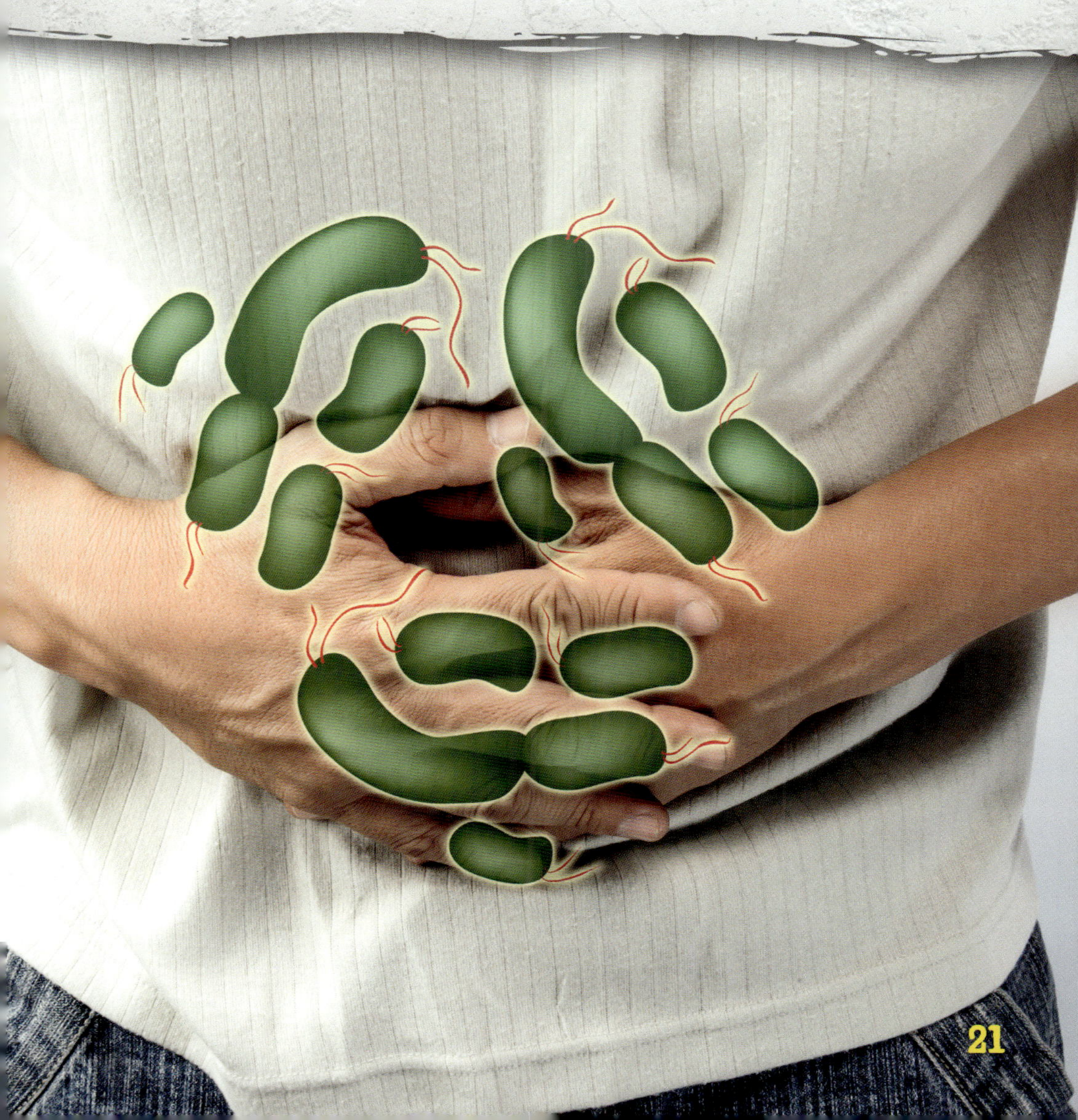

GLOSSARY

asymptomatic – not presenting with signs or symptoms of infection, illness, or disease.

contaminated – infected by contact.

delirious – confused from a high fever.

infect – to spread germs or disease to.

isolation – separation from others to stop spread of disease.

sanitation – providing resources for public health, like clean water and sewage disposal.

transmit – to pass a disease to someone or something else.

vaccine – a medicine or cure to help end or manage an illness within someone.

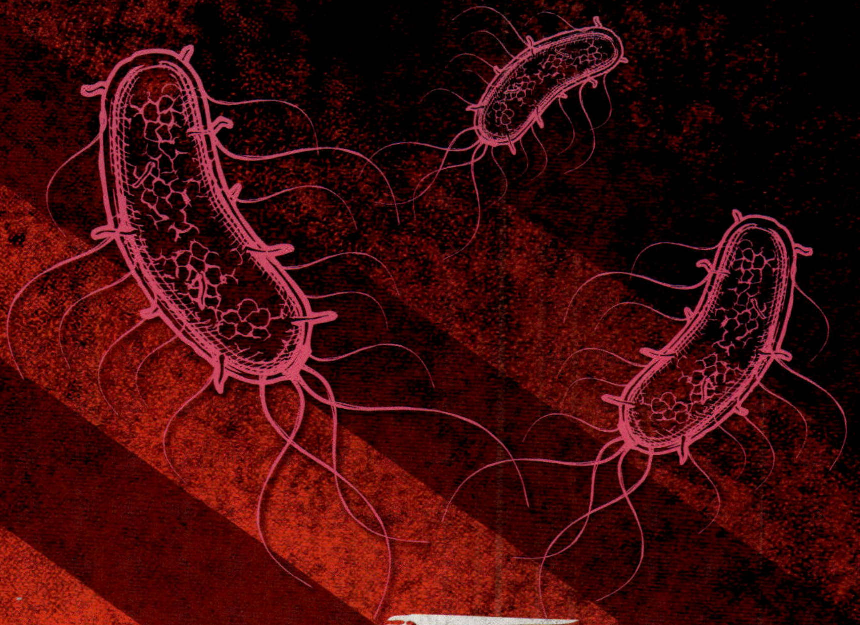

ONLINE RESOURCES

Booklinks
NONFICTION NETWORK
FREE! ONLINE NONFICTION RESOURCES

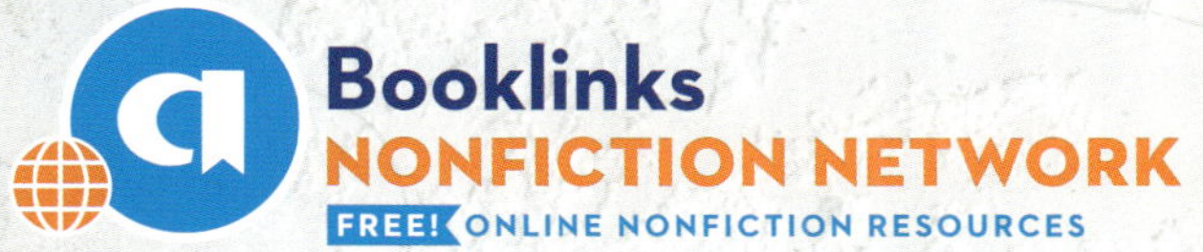

To learn more about Typhoid Epidemic, please visit abdobooklinks.com or scan this QR code. These links are routinely monitored and updated to provide the most current information available.

INDEX

Ireland 14

Mallon, "Typhoid" Mary 6, 14, 15, 16, 17, 18

prevention 21

Salmonella 10

Soper, George 15

spread 10, 13, 15, 16, 17, 18, 21

symptoms 8, 9

treatment 18, 20, 21

United States 14

Warren, Charles 15